I0407852

Happier brain, happier you, happier world
Let's prevent strokes together!
First part

Dr. Ana-Maria Ninulescu

The content of this book is for general instruction only. Each person's physical, emotional, and spiritual condition is unique. The instruction in this book is not intended to replace or interrupt the reader's relationship with a physician or other professional. Please consult your doctor for matters pertaining to your specific health and diet.

To contact the author, visit
fireupgrade.net

Printed in the United States of America

Table of Contents

Introduction

As I begin to write this book, my thoughts go to Mr. B. He was one of my patients.

Aged 52, he lived his whole life trying to make the people around him feel happy and safe. He worked as a guardian at a small cinema.

I can clearly see him in my mind. He was a tall and solid man. In spite of that, some friends would call him "The Little One".

He didn't mind that nickname at all. Actually, he enjoyed being called that, as he always felt that a kid's soul was inside of his big body.

He remembers even now, going fishing with his grandfather as a child. They would laugh a lot and he would learn so many amazing things. After the fishing trip, his grandmother would cook the fish they caught for the entire family at home.

Those were indeed happy days for him. He promised himself that he would do the same thing with his children when they grow up, and also with his grandchildren.

He surely did go on to have fishing trips with his kids and they had an amazing connection. I could clearly see it in their daily interactions.

One day, Mr. B was sent to the hospital after having a stroke. One of his hands would not move at all.

His family was devastated, as anyone else in their place would be. They wanted to know how they could make him feel better and ease his recovery. They naturally had many questions.

There was one particular question that his three sons had. They wanted to know what to do to prevent a stroke from happening to them, too. They were especially worried because Mr B's brother had died several years ago after having a stroke.

Mr. B himself asked me the same question. He was in so much pain at the mere thought that his children may live through such a suffering.

At that moment, I tried my best to explain the situation to them, face to face.

Now, this book, divided into three small pocket-friendly volumes, so it can be easily read and carried, is intended to be a written answer to their burning question. It will also provide answers to anyone aware of the negative effects that a stroke can cause in someone's life, and to those who would like to know how such a terrible disease can be prevented.

Medical research shows that there is a positive correlation between the risk of stroke and certain predictive factors.

We will review these studies together, and by the end of this book, you will know what to do to significantly decrease the risk of having a stroke.

What is a stroke?

Stroke is a condition that appears when the blood flow in the brain is altered either by a hemorrhage or a blockage.

For example, when someone has high blood pressure, a hemorrhage may occur as a result of a blood vessel's rupture.

However, hemorrhagic strokes can appear in various other circumstances as well, for instance, when an aneurysm becomes ruptured.

A hemorrhagic stroke leads to the death of brain cells, and the evolution depends on several factors such as: how big the hemorrhage was, where it was located, whether the evacuation of the blood was possible or not, and what was the general state of health prior to the event.

But hemorrhagic stroke is not the most frequent type of stroke.

The most common strokes are the ischemic ones, or when a clot or another obstructive particle that has traveled to the brain via the arteries blocks the blood flow. This is called an embolus.

So, the obstructive particle may not be only a clot, but also an air bubble, a fat globule, or a fragment of a plaque that was present previously on an artery wall.

Again, the evolution after such a stroke depends on multiple variables, like what artery was blocked, how big it was, where was it located, how fast the blockage disappeared, and, of course, what was the general state of health prior to the event.

Why? Because when blood flow is damaged, the brain cells lack oxygen and nutrients and they die. The number of brain cells affected by this event depends on the variables discussed before and when they die the functions in the brain they were responsible for aren't possible anymore. We perceive this as a deficit.

As an example, if the dead brain cells were involved in locomotion, the injury may translate into the impossibility of moving an arm, a leg, or both. If they were involved in speaking, we are confronted with the impossibility of speaking, also known as aphasia.

Or, we may also observe so-called poststroke dementia. This includes memory problems and other cognitive difficulties in a person who has had no such issues before. It can also include behavioral changes. This happens when the places in the brain involved in controlling memory, cognitive functions, or behavior are affected by the stroke.

As a matter of fact, in a study by Japanese researchers, it was found that the prevalence of dementia was 3% for those without a history of stroke events, and was 27% among stroke survivors. (5)

And, these are only a few examples of what can happen after a stroke; the list of possible symptoms is much longer.

Sometimes, even a small stroke can lead to great changes in a person's thinking and behavior.

I remember a man around 60 years old who had hypertension and diabetes; he didn't take care of these conditions very well.

However, he was feeling well, and mentally speaking, he was in good shape. He still enjoyed playing chess with his friends on the weekends.

Yet one day, he had a small stroke and things changed for him irreversibly. His memory and power of concentration were altered, and also, he'd say things that weren't coherent at times.

I saw both his wife and his son who asked how it was possible to undergo such a poor evolution so quickly, when he was perfectly fine before.

In this case, the problems appeared not because of this event only. It was the combined effect of several subclinical lesions prior to this one. Hypertension and diabetes can lead to this.

Subclinical means that we can't readily observe it. This is because one can have small strokes and not even realize it; and then, even with the addition of another small stroke, major changes can become visible. This is the case in vascular dementia, for example.

Patients or their close ones can easily have the wrong impression that everything is just the way it is supposed to be.

They might think that one is just getting old, but we need to remember that aging is not a disease by itself, and that we can age happily when we take proper care of ourselves.

Is there anything practical we can do?

The natural question that arises when seeing someone suffering from the effects of a stroke is what can we do to prevent this disease from happening to others.

And the good news is that we can actively diminish much of the risk of stroke, by having a healthy lifestyle.

What does this mean? It means not smoking, avoiding excessive alcohol intake, doing regular physical activity, and having a healthy diet.

One's diet should include greens, whole grains, plenty of fruits and vegetables, legumes, nuts, and drinking enough water.

It also means learning to relax and improve one's reaction to stress.

It means sleeping enough and making several lifestyle changes, which together will promote good brain health.

In the next chapters of the book, we will discuss in detail which preventable actions to take, in order to significantly diminish the risk of having a stroke.

There are so many studies that show the importance of lifestyle in preventing strokes.

For example, one is the INTERSTROKE study. Initially, researchers evaluated 6000 people in 22 countries, and their findings suggest that 10 risk factors are associated with 90% of increased risk of stroke.

Those 10 factors are: history of hypertension, current smoking habits, obesity, poor diet, lack of physical activity, diabetes mellitus, excessive alcohol intake (more than 30 drinks per month or binge drinking), psychosocial factors (like stress or depression), cardiac causes and dyslipidemia.

They found that these risk factors are all significant for ischemic stroke, whereas hypertension, smoking, obesity, diet, and alcohol intake were found to be significant risk factors for hemorrhagic stroke. (6)

The second part of the study included another 20,000 people from 32 countries.

This is enough evidence that most strokes are heavily influenced by factors that can be changed.

And the INTERSTROKE study is only one example. There are many other studies that have been conducted to assess the risk factors for stroke, because this is a very debilitating disease and the health costs of treatment and recovery are huge. Not only that, but in too many cases the recovery is only partial, as there are deep physical, emotional and social difficulties that develop after stroke.

We will also speak in detail about some of these studies in the next pages. Together, they prove that the effect of diminishing the risk of stroke stands true. Tens of thousands of people were included in some of these studies, and hundreds of thousands in others. After the results were analyzed, conclusions were drawn that our bodies react similarly to the main risk factors.

What does this mean?

It means that we can do a lot to prevent a stroke. It is definitely not a disease written in our genes, which will happen no matter what.

Yes, there are some particular situations and some rare diseases that predispose people to having a stroke, it is true. But here, we are going to speak about how to prevent the majority of strokes, knowing full well that when we are in prevention mode, we are actively and significantly diminishing the risk of having a stroke, not completely erasing the risk. However, significantly diminishing this risk is also extremely important.

And even when one has a rare disease that might increase the risk of having a stroke, one can also benefit from applying the lifestyle changes we are going to talk about in the next chapters, because they are targeted towards maintaining a healthy cardiovascular system and a healthy brain, both of which are proven to increase life expectancy and overall well-being.

What about my Uncle Joe, doc?

I know that sometimes we tend to notice the exceptions we see in our lives. These are people who lived a long life and did things proven to shorten one's lifespan; and yet, they somehow managed to cheat the statistics and live long and well.

Let's call them "Uncle Joes".

Yes, these kinds of people do exist, but they are, as I said before, exceptions. Most of us don't resist like that.

The studies prove it. They don't say that everybody who smokes will have a stroke, but they do say that smokers tend to have more strokes, and at a younger age.

The reality is that our bodies are rather frail, even if we don't like to admit it. That's why we should take good care of ourselves.

As I say this, I'm thinking about someone who used to smoke, someone I knew well. When I would tell him that he is risking his life doing that, he'd always say the same thing: that his father lived to be 83 years old, and when he died, the cause was not related to smoking. To make a long story short, he did quit smoking, one week before dying of terminal lung cancer at 64.

The image of his devastated children at his funeral will forever remain a very sad memory of mine.

Since then, I decided to become an active supporter who helps people quit smoking.

And I personally know that people have many regrets when they get sick because they kept doing something that was harming their bodies.

These are behaviors that they could have stopped, but they just didn't. As a matter of fact, when a lethal disease appears, the regrets are amplified, but there rarely is something practical one can do to reverse it. Regrets alone don't help.

Generally, we tend to think that nothing bad will happen to ourselves, that it is always other people who become ill. And when it happens to us, it is, for many, shocking.

You know, I have nothing against positive thinking; I am all for it. But, when we have positive ideas regarding our health while we do harmful things to our body, we may simply be avoiding reality and living in incongruence.

As a matter of fact, positive thinking and harmful actions are not a good combination, and may be much more dangerous than one can imagine.

And you know what? When looking at the lives of those so-called exceptions, we don't really know how much longer they would have lived if that unhealthy habit had not existed. The sister of the person I was speaking before is 85, and is in a very good shape for her age. And their father, the one who lived to be 83 as a smoker, before his death he said that he would have wanted to live longer.

Actually, it is not just him who says that; we all know that in the face of death, most people would like to live a little longer, as one's life ahead is still desirable at any age, while the past seems to have been condensed into short moments.

I used to ask my grandfather what it is like to live 80 plus years; he'd always blink twice with his eyes and say, "just like that".

And I remember that I once had a patient, a lovely lady also aged 80 plus. She had a cancer several years ago. She completed a treatment that was successful at the time, but now the cancer had come back.

When talking to her, she confessed to me that she was grateful for the life she had. It was a long and beautiful one.

She understood her health problems perfectly, but said that she would just love to live 5 more months to attend her grandson's wedding.

These stories are why I feel that it is so important to write a book about preventable risk factors that can rob our lives not of months, but of many years. And I will not say "just" months, because there is no such thing such as "just" months. Every minute is important.

Nowadays we want to live a long life and as healthy as possible. But in order to do that, is not sufficient to see modern medicine as something that will make us healthy again no matter what; we also need to know and apply the principles of self-caring and prevention of diseases.

And if this is the case, let's see how we can practically prevent strokes, increase our life expectancy and improve our overall well-being.

The Big Question

What is good for us, what is bad, and what is really damaging?

We often find ourselves asking these kinds of questions, as contradictory information keeps coming into our lives.

We might often feel at a loss, not knowing where to start, what to avoid, and what to indulge in.

To make things even more difficult, some theories are elaborated by people who draw their conclusions from their own life experience, and those conclusions may not be valid for everybody, as one person's body may react in one way to certain circumstances, while another may react in a very different way to the same circumstances.

We might then feel that something is wrong with us, that we are somehow broken and that there is no possible solution to make us whole again.

In these situations, I find it best to refer to medical studies that have been conducted on the subject we are interested in.

For example, there is this egg debate. Almost everyone knows that eggs contain cholesterol and that many people do not encourage their consumption. This is based on the fact that, due to their cholesterol content, their ingestion is supposed to increase the risk of cardiovascular disease. I know people who stay away from eggs based on this assumption.

Now, research has been conducted to see whether this is true, and some new studies show that moderate egg consumption may actually be beneficial.

For example, the analysis of egg consumption and carotid atherosclerosis in the Northern Manhattan Study concluded that low to moderate egg consumption in healthy people is not associated with an increase in the carotid atherosclerosis, and that it is not associated with an increase in stroke incidence or other clinical vascular events. Therefore, this analysis doesn't support that avoiding egg consumption will promote vascular health. (1)

Also, a meta-analysis concluded that the intake of up to 1 egg daily may be associated with reduced risk of total stroke. (2)

Why? Because eggs contain lots of nutrients like vitamins, minerals, proteins, lecithin and other compounds that can result in beneficial effects.

However, another study found that in men, daily egg consumption of one or more eggs a day, with a total of 7 or more eggs a week was associated with a 30% higher risk of heart failure, while eating 6 eggs a week or less was not associated with this condition. (3)

And another meta-analysis found out that those who eat 1 egg per day or more, each day of the week, are 42% more likely to develop type 2 diabetes. And, that among diabetic patients, frequent egg consumers (1 egg per day or more) are 69% more likely to have cardiovascular problems. (4)

These studies remind me of my neighbor, who came to me one day very enthusiastically, and told me that he heard on TV how eggs are good for health, and that he was planning to eat an 8 egg omelet for dinner.

I tried to explain to him how that was not going to improve his health, on the contrary.

While some people are egg intolerant, as they cannot consume eggs at all, others may benefit from moderately consuming them. The key word here is moderation.

So, in this particular case, studies have shown that eating 4 to 5 eggs a week is not dangerous for healthy people.

Do not eat all of the eggs in one day, of course. Moderation, again, is key.

Me, for healthy people, I personally recommend a vegan menu at least 2 days a week and moderate consumption of animal protein during the rest of the week. I recommend at least one week of a completely vegan menu every 3 months.

In the chapter dedicated to nutrition, we will talk more about egg consumption, vegetarianism, and other very interesting topics.

The conclusions drawn from medical studies can allow someone understand the importance of a healthy lifestyle and add healthy changes to their daily program. The consideration that something is harmful for thousands and tens of thousands of people is pretty convincing, right?

Also, because I know that often adding healthy habits into our life and removing the bad ones might be difficult to do alone, I support health coaching, and I incorporate it into my practice.

Why? Because health coaching provides you with a program and a support system from a certified health coach, who is by your side on this journey.

I, for example, provide a renewable 6 month program of nutritional health coaching for those who want to quit smoking, but are afraid to gain weight. This is accomplished with a 50 minute session every 2 weeks, in which I consistently support my clients to achieve the best results in the context of their life. I offer the first session for free to see if we are a good fit for each other.

Having compatibility between the health coach and the client is fundamental to achieving good results.

Of course, you can find more about my practice on my website.

Now, returning to this book, why did I write it?

Because I want you to know how you can protect yourself from having a stroke, and I also want you to actively begin the steps to achieve this goal.

Together, in the next pages we will discuss about these preventable risk factors in detail, so that you can do your best to take care of your health.

Preventable cardiac causes of stroke

Hypertension is definitely a risk factor for stroke, both hemorrhagic and ischemic.

It is one of many diseases that can remain silent for years. This means that one may have it and not be aware of its presence, so the simplest practical step we can accomplish to diminish the risk of stroke and take care of the overall health is to periodically check one's blood pressure.

If hypertension is not properly treated, the quality of the blood vessels is altered by and by, and the small arteries all over the body are slowly damaged. This creates complications in the brain when the brain's small vessels are damaged, or hypertensive retinopathy when the vessels of the eye are damaged, and many other complications in various other organs.

But this is not the only cardiac cause of strokes.

One of the most common cardiac causes for ischemic stroke is atrial fibrillation.

In this case, the heart loses its ability to contract rhythmically; it becomes irregular, having less force of contraction. The blood pools inside the heart, clots are formed, and, at a particular moment, parts of the clots may move into the blood stream and block an artery in the brain.

That's why having an irregular pulse is always a sign of concern, and needs to be investigated immediately by a cardiologist.

Other cardiac causes for ischemic strokes might include: atrial mixoma, valvular heart disease, endocarditis, and myocardial infarction.

All of these conditions require medical treatment and careful surveillance from a cardiologist.

That being said, is absolutely standard to have cardiologists from all over the world involved in stroke prevention.

For example, the American Heart Association came with "Life's Simple 7". These are 7 key health factors and behaviors that diminish risks for heart disease and stroke. They also came with the 2020 goal plan: to improve the cardiovascular health of all Americans by 20 percent and reduce deaths from cardiovascular diseases and stroke by 20 percent, by the year 2020.

Life's Simple 7 are:

- not smoking,
- physical activity,
- healthy diet,
- body weight,
- control of cholesterol, blood pressure and blood sugar.

Some of the epidemiologic data they gathered look like this:

- In 2010, worldwide prevalence of stroke was 33 million, with 16.9 million people having a first stroke.
- Stroke kills someone in the U.S. about once every 4 minutes.
- Someone in the U.S. has a stroke about once every 40 seconds.
- Stroke is the leading preventable cause of disability. (7)

A woman once came to see me. She was around 60 years old, and had been previously diagnosed with hypertension. She told me that she was not taking the prescribed pills because she was not feeling sick, that her body became accustomed to the high tensional values, and that she had no problem with it. Plus, she read the notice and saw that there were so many side effects of the pills; she got sick only by reading about them.

The reality in this case is that, hypertension is not a painful disease; once in the body, it generally remains there even if we have the impression that everything is ok. And it damages the entire body very slowly.

The side effects of the antihypertensive drugs might be scary for some, but many times, these side effects don't happen. And if a side effect occurs, there are so many types of antihypertensive drugs today, that a doctor can replace them immediately with another that is better tolerated.

The effects of untreated hypertension are generally more serious than the side effects of the antihypertensive drugs. You know, untreated hypertension may lead to many complications like palsy, kidney failure and even death.

Yes, I met several persons that were on antihypertensive drugs for a while, and then they didn't need it anymore; but, those are rare cases and they stopped the medication after several visits to the cardiologist and serious examination. It was not something they did by themselves. And generally, this happened to people who worked on changing their lifestyle to a healthier one.

And while it is very important to emphasize that a person diagnosed with hypertension does benefit a lot by applying lifestyle changes like Life's Simple 7, it is also important to emphasize that they do not substitute the medical treatment recommended by the cardiologist.

The most important thing is the association between the lifestyle changes on one hand and the medical treatment on the other hand. One does not substitute the other.

Taking the pills does not mean that it is okay to forget about taking care of ourselves the rest of the time. The sooner we start taking care of ourselves, the better, because otherwise, the overall damage that unhealthy lifestyle causes in our bodies may become irreversible.

In practice, we see that people come to understand this, and they add these recommendations to their life more and more often nowadays.

Now, I can remember a woman who was on daily medication and who added many healthy changes to her lifestyle. In the meantime, her husband teased her about it, but she remained firm on her position and went on with the medical recommendations concerning both her medical treatment and lifestyle changes. Several years later, her husband felt sick. He went for a medical check-up, and received the bad news that his health was so deteriorated, that no medical treatment was possible for him anymore, only painkillers.

He apologized to his wife for his behavior, telling her that he would perform all the lifestyle changes in the world, and take all the pills a doctor would recommend him, just to live a little more. He died shortly afterward.

Good foods versus bad foods

Many studies were conducted to reveal which are the foods that increase the risk of stroke, and which ones diminish it.

For example, there are studies that found long term daily consumption of **red meat** increasing the risk of ischemic stroke, with a greater increase in risk for **processed meat**. Perhaps this is because of the sodium content in this type of meat and of the contained additives. (8)(9) (10) (11)(12) (13) (14) (15) (16)

One meta-analysis that studied dietary patterns and their influence on the risk of stroke, based on studies that followed the dietary patterns of people for many years, found that there was a significant increase of ischemic stroke risk for each increase in serving per day of fresh red meat, processed meat, and total red meat consumption, one serving being equal to 50 g of processed meat and 100-120 g of fresh red meat and total red meat. (12)

I personally believe that the long term daily consumption of red meat is not the best thing we can do for our health.

And it is not only me that thinks like that. The working group of the International Agency for Research on Cancer (IARC), the cancer agency of the World Health Organization, has classified the consumption of red meat as probably carcinogenic (Group 2A).

This association was mainly observed for colorectal cancer, but also for pancreatic cancer and prostate cancer as well.

Additionally, processed meat was classified as carcinogenic (Group 1), based on sufficient evidence that the consumption of processed meat causes colorectal cancer. (17)

Plus, there are studies that found that each serving per day of processed meat was associated with a higher risk of coronary heart disease and a higher risk of diabetes mellitus. (18)

And what do we do now that we know about it? How do we apply this information to our lives?

While for some it is very easy to diminish and even eliminate red meat from their diets, for others it is very difficult.

However, **flexitarianism** may be a good option for many.

This is a term for a trend that has appeared recently. It is mainly a vegetarian diet, with fish or meat added now and then.

The good news is that flexitarianism seems to have beneficial effects on health. (19)

And it looks like there is a growing number of flexitarians all over the world.

Also, substituting poultry, fish, whole-fat diary, low-fat dairy and nuts for red meat was associated with a lower stroke risk. (15)

Regarding **milk and its derivatives**, several studies were conducted to assess their effects on cardiovascular health, but the results are contradictory. More research seems to be needed in this area. (20) (21) (22) (23) (24)

Fermented milk appears to have a role in decreasing the progression of atherosclerotic disease, in some studies starting even from 100g/day. (25) (26)

Of course, those who are lactose intolerant need to stay away from milk and derivates.

And while the studies about meat and stroke risk might be useful for omnivores, we cannot help but see an increasing number of **vegans and vegetarians** all around the world.

Vegetarians don't consume meat at all, and vegans don't consume any animal product; they don't eat eggs, and they don't eat dairy.

Now, what is it about these diets? Does a vegan diet come with health advantages?

Some studies have focused on the gut microbiome, or the germs that live in our intestines. Those germs are implied in digestion; but, they also might be linked to the overall health of a person, as new studies are showing.

In this direction, research was conducted to assess the differences between the vegan gut microbiome and the gut microbiome of vegetarians and omnivores. It seems that the vegan and vegetarian microbiome are not always significantly different; but, there is a difference between the vegans' and omnivores' microbiomes, with the vegan microbiome having fewer dangerous germs and greater protective species, which can be linked with reduced levels of inflammation. (27)

At the same time, a high risk of having a stroke is correlated with a high level of inflammation.

Oxidative stress and chronic inflammation are seen also in hypertension, atrial fibrillation, diabetes, smoking, chronic excessive alcohol intake, atherosclerosis and other conditions and situations that increase the risk of stroke. (28) (29) (30) (31) (32) (33) (34)

That's why it is important that, in our pursuit of diminishing the risk of stroke, to also aim to diminish inflammation and oxidative stress. How? Well, one of the most effective ways of doing this is through alimentation. (35) (36) (37) (38) (39) (40)

Normally, the healthy body has the capacity to come with compensatory mechanisms and maintain equilibrium; but, with time, when we use and overuse those mechanisms, they become less and less effective.

One study sought to reveal what impact a high fat and/or high salt diet could have on the oxidative stress in the heart muscle. An increase in enzymes showed that the normal heart can use compensatory mechanisms to prevent oxidative damage. (41)

But, the situation changes when the oxidative stress increase happens in an organ that is already damaged. (41) (42)

I remember a friend of mine who told me, when we were around 25 years old, that her parents taught her to eat all the red and processed meat and butter and sweets she could before turning 30, because after that she will get sick anyway and she will not be able to eat them anymore. They said that doctors would forbid her from indulging in such behaviors.

They knew it very well, as this was what happened to them.

But, to be honest, this happened to them when they were around 40 years of age. Now, they saw that there was a trend towards getting sick at a younger and younger age. For example, their parents, my friend's grandparents that is, got sick, but at well over 60 years of age. So, they thought that their daughter would get sick around 30, and that she didn't have much time to enjoy life as they understood enjoying life.

And while, for some families, the reality might be that their members tend to get sick at younger ages than their parents and grandparents, it happens usually because of the changes in the lifestyle, one notable change being the change in the eating habits.

Nowadays we tend to add greater amounts of foods that increase oxidative stress and inflammation. Therefore, we are going to solve this problem not by overeating these foods while we are still young and "can", but by limiting their intake, no matter what age, so that we don't damage the compensatory mechanisms built within our bodies.

The same is the case with the microbiome. It slowly changes in accordance with what we eat. Sometimes those changes can further increase the oxidative stress and inflammation.

For example, we have talked about the egg debate in the beginning of the book. Some say that eggs are bad for health, while others say they are not. In reality everything depends on quantity, as we saw, and it also depends on personal metabolism.

Why? Well, this is one of those cases in which the gut microbiome is tremendously important in the way the egg is digested in our body.

You know, from eggs and several other animal sources, metabolites can be formed in the gut that are related to an increase in atherosclerosis and thrombosis, which can lead to all kinds of cardiovascular problems, including heart attack and stroke. (43) (46)

Those metabolites are formed in the gut, by special types of germs that live there.

Now, if we don't have too many germs like that, we can eat eggs without having those metabolites in our blood stream at high levels. While if we have those germs, we can have high values of these metabolites in the blood stream even from one small egg.

For example, one of those molecules, called TMAO, was related with an increase of atherosclerosis and thrombosis.

Furthermore, studies showed that there are people who are high TMAO producers and low TMAO producers, meaning that with the same meal, some people produce more of it, while others less, all depending on their microbiota.(43)

And the gut microbiota, in turn, is highly dependent on what we eat. For example, the germs that produce a great quantity of TMAO are developed through a diet high in carbohydrates, red and processed meat. (45)

Vegans and vegetarians produce less TMAO than omnivorous people, following the ingestion of the same dose of L-carnitine, a compound found in red meat. (46)

So, not only are we are slowly damaging our health because of the direct effect of the food components and metabolites by eating specific products, but we favor the development of gut microbiota that will in turn increase the inflammation, oxidative stress and the risk of systemic atherosclerosis from the by-products of gut metabolism. (47)

That's why in the case of the persons already diagnosed with cardiovascular diseases and diabetes mellitus, it is best to eat less than 200 mg of cholesterol per day, diminish the intake of processed meat, and favor vegetarian eating habits. Many times, their microbiota is already modified at the moment of diagnosis, so we should pay great attention to what we are feeding those germs as well. (44)

Conclusions

Stroke is a major disability cause in our modern society. It can lead to palsy, memory problems, behavioral changes, death.

This book, divided into three small pocket-friendly volumes is intended to provide answers to those who would like to know how such a terrible disease can be prevented.

It is not enough to see modern medicine as something that will make us healthy again no matter what; we also need to know and apply the principles of self-caring and prevention of diseases. The reality is that we can actively diminish much of the risk of stroke, just by having a healthy lifestyle.

The conclusions of medical studies can allow someone understand the importance of a healthy lifestyle and add healthy changes to their daily program. The consideration that something is harmful for thousands and tens of thousands of people is pretty convincing, right?

It is also very important to know how our bodies react and what they specifically need in order to stay healthy, as one person's body may react in one way to certain circumstances, while another may react in a very different way to the same circumstances.

But, no matter the individual differences, there are some main areas we should all pay attention to.

We covered in this volume some of those areas, such as the cardiovascular risk factors, we evaluated some nutritional aspects of preventing strokes, and we analyzed the new trend called flexitarianism, and the new findings regarding the microbiota.

Which are the takeaway points?

Well, we should never forget that **hypertension** is definitely a risk factor for stroke, both hemorrhagic and ischemic.

We should keep in mind that this is one of many diseases that can remain silent for years. This means that one may have it and not be aware of it, so the simplest practical step we can accomplish to diminish the risk of stroke and take care of the overall health is to periodically check one's blood pressure and treat it if it's higher than normal.

In the case of hypertension, like in the case of many other diseases, the association between the lifestyle changes on one hand and the medical treatment on the other hand is crucial. One does not substitute the other.

As we previously discussed, taking the pills does not mean that it is okay to forget about taking care of ourselves the rest of the time. The sooner we start taking care of ourselves, the better, because otherwise, the overall damage that unhealthy lifestyle causes in our bodies may become irreversible.

Another risk factor for stroke we have talked about is long term daily consumption of **red meat**. It increases the risk of ischemic stroke. **Processed meat** increases it even more. Processed meat was also classified as carcinogenic, based on the evidence that it causes colorectal cancer.

We have also covered the fact that **fermented milk** appears to have a role in decreasing the progression of the atherosclerotic disease, in some studies starting even from 100g/day.

We reviewed why **flexitarianism** may be a good option for many and why the types of germs in the gut are very important for our health.

But our journey is just beginning. New studies and new information will be covered in the next two parts. We will talk about body weight and whole foods, vitamins and minerals, the fat controversy, water, emotions, noise, music, smoking, alcohol and their effects on the brain.

In the final volume, we will concentrate on developing **a 12 week program** focused on significantly decreasing the risk of having a stroke. We will start with simple steps that can have a major influence on our brain health and overall wellness.

But first, we will cover the why, and then the how.

In the meantime, if you want a free online consultation, just stop by my website (fireupgrade.net) and send me a message. I will be so glad to talk to you!

Thanks for being with me on this journey!

About the Author

Dr Ana-Maria Ninulescu is a specialist in geriatrics with a passion for nutrition and disease prevention.

She enjoys coaching people to a better health and happy aging.

Recently, she has developed a new program for those who want to quit smoking, but are afraid of weight gain, called the Fireupgrade method. By the way, smoking is also significantly increasing the risk of stroke, as you will see in the next volumes.

For more information, you can find her at fireupgrade.net.

References:

1. Sharon Goldberg, Hannah Gardener, Eduard Tiozzo, Cheung Ying Kuen, Mitchell SV Elkind, Ralph L Sacco, Tatjana Rudenk. Egg Consumption and Carotid Atherosclerosis in the Northern Manhattan Study. Atherosclerosis. 2014 Aug:235(2): 273-280.

2. Alexander DD, Miller PE, Vargas AJ, Weed DL, Cohen SS. Meta-analysis of Egg Consumption and Risk of Coronary Heart Disease and Stroke. J Am Coll Nutr 2016 Nov-Dec;35(8):704-716. Epub 2016 Oct 6.

3. Larsson Sc, Akesson A, Wolk A. Egg consumption and risk of heart failure, myocardial infarction, and stroke: results from 2 prospective cohorts. Am J Clin Nutr 2015 Nov;102(5):1007-1013. doi: 10.3945/ajcn.115.119263. Epub 2015 Sep 23.

4. Jang Yel Shin, PengCheng Xun, Yasuyuki Nakamura, Ka He. Egg consumption in relation to risk of cardiovascular disease and diabetes: a systematic review and meta-analysis. Am J Clin Nutr 2013 Jul; 98(1): 146–159. Published online 2013 May 15. doi: 10.3945/ajcn.112.051318.

5. Nagata K, Suzuki K. Update on stroke epidemiology. Brain Nerve 2013 Jul;65(7):857-70.

6. Martin J O'Donnel, Denis Xavier, Lisheng Liu, Hongye Zhang, Siu Lim Chin, Purnima Rao-Melacini, Sumathy Rangarajan, Shofiqul Islam, Prem Pais, Matthew J Mc Queen, Charles Mondo, Albertino Damasceno, Patricio Lopez-Jaramillo, Graeme J Hankey, Antonio L Dans, Khalid Yusoff, Thomas Truelsen, Hans-Christoph Diener, Ralph L Sacco, Danuta Ryglewicz, Anna Czlonkowska, Christian Weimar, Xingyu Wang, salim Yusuf, D Phil. Risk factors for ischaemic and intracerebral haemorrhagic stroke in 22 countries (the

INTERSTROKE study): a case-control study . The Lancet 2010 Jul; 9735(376), 112-123.

7. Mozaffarian D, Benjamin EJ, Go AS, Arnett DK, Blaha MJ, Cushman M, Das SR, de Ferranti S, Després J-P, Fullerton HJ, Howard VJ, Huffman MD, Isasi CR, Jiménez MC, Judd SE, Kissela BM, Lichtman JH, Lisabeth LD, Liu S, Mackey RH, Magid DJ, McGuire DK, Mohler ER III, Moy CS, Muntner P, Mussolino ME, Nasir K, Neumar RW, Nichol G, Palaniappan L, Pandey DK, Reeves MJ, Rodriguez CJ, Rosamond W, Sorlie PD, Stein J, Towfighi A, Turan TN, Virani SS, Woo D, Yeh RW, Turner MB; on behalf of the American Heart Association Statistics Committee and Stroke Statistics Subcommittee. Heart disease and stroke statistics—2016 update: a report from the American Heart Association [published online ahead of print December 16, 2015]. Circulation. doi: 10.1161/CIR.0000000000000350. **Circulation.** 2016;133:447-454, originally published January 25, 2016.

8. Yang C, Pan L, Xi Y, Li D. Red Meat Consumption and the Risk of Stroke: A Dose-Response Meta-analysis of Prospective Cohort Studies. J Stroke Cerebrovasc Dis 2016 May;25(5):1177-86. doi: 10.1016/j.jstrokecerebrovasdis.2016.01.040. Epub 2016 Feb 27.

9. Shay CM, Stamler J, Dyer AR, Brown IJ, Chan Q, Elliott P, Zhao L, Okuda N, Miura K, Daviglus ML, Van Horn L. Nutrient and food intakes of middle-aged adults at low risk of cardiovascular disease: the international study of macro-/micronutrients and blood pressure (INTERMAP). Eur J Nutr 2012 Dec;51(8):917-26. doi: 10.1007/s00394-011-0268-2. Epub 2011 Nov 6.

10. Battaglia Richi E, Baumer B, Conrad B, Darioli R, Schmid A, Keller U. Health Risks Associated with Meat Consumption: A Review of Epidemiological Studies. Int J Vitam Nutr Res 2015;85(1-2):70-8. doi: 10.1024/0300-9831/a000224.

11. Renata Micha, Sarah K Wallace, Darius Mozaffarian. Red and processed meat consumption and risk of incident coronary heart disease, stroke, and diabetes: A systematic review and meta-analysis. Circulation 2010 Jun 1: 121 (21): 2271-2283. doi: 10.1161/CIRCULATIONAHA.109.924977.

12. Joanna Kaluza, Alicja Wolk, Susanna C Larsson. Red meat consumption and risk of stroke: a meta-analysis of prospective studies. Stroke 2012;43:2556-2560. doi: 10.1161/STROKEAHA.112.663286.

13. Susanna C Larsson, Jarmo Virtamo, Alicja Wolk. Red Meat Consumption and Risk of Stroke in Swedish Women. Stroke 2011;42:324-329. Doi: 10.1161/STROKEAHA.110.596510.

14. Susanna C Larsson, Jarmo Virtamo, Alicja Wolk. Red Meat Consumption and Risk of Stroke in Swedish Men. Am J Clin Nutr August 2011 vol. 94 no. 2 417-421. doi: 10.3945/ajcn.111.015115.

15. Adam M Bernstein, An Pan, Kathryn M Rexrode, Meir Stampfer, Frank B Hu, Dariush Mozaffarian, Walter C Willett. Dietary Protein Sources and the Risk of Stroke in Men and Women. Stroke 2012;43:637-644. doi: 10.1161/STROKEAHA.111.633404.

16. Chen GC, Lv DB, Pang Z, Liu QF. Red and processed meat consumption and risk of stroke: a meta-analysis of prospective cohort studies. Red and processed meat consumption and risk of stroke: a meta-analysis of prospective cohort studies. Eur J Clin Nutr 2013 Jan:67(1):91-5. doi:10.1038/ejcn.2012.180. Epub 2012 Nov 21.

17. Véronique Bouvard, Dana Loomis, Kathryn Z Guyton, Yann Grosse, Fatiha El Ghissassi, Lamia Benbrahim-Tallaa, Neela Guha, Heidi Mattock, Kurt Straif on behalf of the International Agency for Research on Cancer Monograph Working Group. Carcinogenicity of consumption of red and processed meat. The Lancet Oncology 2015 Dec 16 (16): 1599-1600.

18. Renata Micha, Sarah K Wallace, Darius Mozaffarian. Red and processed meat consumption and risk of incident coronary heart disease, stroke, and diabetes: A systematic review and meta-analysis. Circulation 2010 Jun 1: 121 (21): 2271-2283. doi: 10.1161/CIRCULATIONAHA.109.924977.

19. Emma J Derbyshire. Flexitarian Diets and Health: A Review of the Evidence-Based Literature. Front Nutr 2016 3:55. Doi: 10.3389/fnut.2016.00055.

20. Elwood PC, Pickering JE, Hughes J, Fehily AM, NessAR. Milk drinking, ischaemic heart disease and ischaemic stroke II. Evidence from cohort studies. Eur J Clin Nutr 2004 May;58(5):718-24.

21. Mohammad Y Yakoob, Peilin Shi, Frank B u, Hannia Campos, Kathryn M Rexrode, E John Oray, walter C Willett, Dariush Mozaffarian. Circulating biomarkers of dairy fat and risk of incident stroke in U.S. men and women in 2 large prospective cohorts. Am J Clin Nutr 2014 Dec; 100(6): 1437-1447. doi: 10.3945/ajcn.114.083097.

22. Janette de Goede, Sabita S Soedamah-Muthu, An Pan, Lieke Gijsbers, Johanna M Geleijnse. Dairy Consumption and Risk of Stroke: A Systematic Review and Updated Dose–Response Meta-Analysis of Prospective Cohort Studies. J Am Heart Assoc 2016 May; 5(5): e002787.

23. Beth H Rice. Dairy and Cardiovascular Disease: A Review of Recent Observational Research. Curr Nutr Rep 2014; 3(2): 130-138. Doi: 10.1007/s13668-014-0076-4

24. Tanja Kongerslev Thorning, Anne Raben, tine Tholstrup, Sabita S Soedamah-Muthu, Ian Givens, Arne Astrup. Milk and dairy products: good or bad for human health? An assessment of the totality of scientific evidence. Food Nutr Res 2016; 60: 10.3402/fnr.v60.32527. doi: 10.3402/fnr.v60.32527.

25. Kerry L Ivey, Joshua R Lewis, Jonathan M Hodgson, Kun Zhu, Satvinder S Dhaliwal, Peter L Thompson, Richard L Prince. Association between yogurt, milk and cheese consumption and common carotid artery intima-media thickness and cardiovascular disease risk factors in elderly women. *Am J Clin Nutr* July 2011; 94(1): 234-239. doi: 10.3945/ajcn.111.014159.

26. Glick-Bauer M, Yeh MC. The health advantage of a vegan diet: exploring the gut microbiota connection. Nutrients 2014 Oct 31; 6(11):4822-38. doi: 10.3390/nu6114822.

27. Da Silva RM. Influence of Inflammation and Atherosclerosis in Atrial Fibrillation. Curr Atheroscler Rep 2017 Jan;19(1):2. doi: 10.1007/s11883-017-0639-0.

28. Giannopoulos G, Cleman MMW, Deftereos S. Inflammation fueling atrial fibrillation substrate: seeking ways to "cool" the heart. Med Chem 2014;10(7):663-71.

29. Van Wagoner DR. Oxidative stress and inflammation in atrial fibrillation: role in pathogenesis and potential as a therapeutic target. J Cardiovasc Pharmacol. 2008 Oct;52(4):306-13. doi: 10.1097/FJC.0b013e31817f9398.

30. Patel P, Dokainish H, Tsai P, Lakkis N. Update on the association of inflammation and atrial fibrillation. J CArdiovasc Electrophysiol. 2010 Sep;21(9):1064-70. doi: 10.1111/j.1540-8167.2010.01774.x.

31. De Ciuceis C, Agabiti-Rosei C, Airo P, Scarsi M, Tincani A, Tiberio GA, Piantoni S, Porteri E, Solaini L, Duse S, Semeraro F, Petroboni B, Mori L, Castellano M, Gavazzi A, Agabiti-Rosei E, Rizzoni D. Relationship between different subpopulations of circulating CD4+ T lymphocytes and microvascular or systemic oxidative stress in humans. Blood Press. 2017 Feb 15:1-9. doi: 10.1080/08037051.2017.1292395.

32. Ahuja M, Buabeid M, Abdel-Rehman E, Majrashi M, Parameshwaran K, Amin R, Ramesh S, thiruchelvan K, Pondugula S, Suppiramaniam V, Dhanasekaran M. Immunological alteration & toxic molecular inductions leading to cognitive impairment & neurotoxicity in transgenic mouse model of Alzheimer's disease. Life Sci 2017 Mar 9. pii: S0024-3205(17)30087-5. doi: 10.1016/j.lfs.2017.03.004. [Epub ahead of print]

33. Bastard JP, Maachi M, Lagathu C, Kim MJ, Caron M, Vidal H, Capeau J, Feve B. Recent advances in the relationship between obesity, inflammation, and insulin resistance. Eur Cytokine Netw. 2006 Mar;17(1):4-12.

34. Hansaem Choe, Ji-Yun Hwang, Jin A Yun, Ji-Myung Kim, Tae-Jin Song, Namsoo Chang, Yong-Jae Kim, Yuri Kim. Intake of antioxidants and B vitamins is inversely associated with ischemic stroke and cerebral atherosclerosis. Nutr Res Pract. 2016 Oct; 10(5): 516–523. Doi: 10.4162/nrp.2016.10.5.516.

35. Vokó Z, Hollander M, Hofman A, Koudstaal PJ, Breteler M. Dietary antioxidants and the risk of ischemic stroke: the Rotterdam Study. Neurology. 2003 Nov 11;61(9):1273-5.

36. Van Guelpen B, Hultdin J, Johansson I, Stegmayr B, Hallmans G, Nilsson TK, Weinehall L, Witthöft C, Palmqvist R, Winkvist A. Folate, vitamin B12, and risk of ischemic and hemorrhagic stroke: a prospective, nested case-referent study of plasma concentrations and dietary intake. Stroke. 2005 Jul;36(7):1426-31. Epub 2005 Jun 2.

37. Larsson SC, Männistö S, Virtanen MJ, Kontto J, Albanes D, Virtamo J. Folate, vitamin B6, vitamin B12, and methionine intakes and risk of stroke subtypes in male smokers. Am J Epidemiol. 2008 Apr 15;167(8):954-61. doi: 10.1093/aje/kwm395. Epub 2008 Feb 12.

38. C R Gale, CN Martyn, PD Winter, C Cooper. Vitamin C and risk of death from stroke and coronary heart disease in cohort of elderly people. BMJ 1995 Jun 17; 319 (6994): 1563–1566.

39. Weng LC, Yeh WT, Bai CH, Chen HJ, Chuang SY, Chang HY, Lin BF, Chen KJ, Pan WH. Is ischemic stroke risk related to folate status or other nutrients correlated with folate intake? Stroke. 2008 Dec;39(12):3152-8. doi: 10.1161/STROKEAHA.108.524934. Epub 2008 Nov 6.

40. Mayyas F, Alzoubi KH, Al-Taleb Z. Impact of high fat/high salt diet on myocardial oxidative stress. Clin Exp Hypertens. 2017;39(2):126-132. doi: 10.1080/10641963.2016.1226894. Epub 2017 Feb 28.

41. Dornas WC, de Lima WG, dos Santos RC, Guerra JF, de Souza MO, Silva M, Soliza e Silva L, Diniz MF, Silva ME. High dietary salt decreases antioxidant defenses in the liver of fructose-fed insulin-resistant rats. J Nutr Biochem. 2013 Dec;24(12):2016-22. doi: 10.1016/j.jnutbio.2013.06.006. Epub 2013 Oct 14.

42. Zeneng Wang, W H Wilson Tang, Jennifer A Buffa, Xiaoming Fu, Earl B Britt, Robert A Koeth, Bruce S Levison, YiYing Fan, Yuping Wu, Stanley L Hazen. Prognostic value of choline and betaine depends on intestinal microbiota-generated metabolite trimethylamine-N-oxide. Eur Heart J. 2014 Apr 7; 35(14): 904–910. doi: 10.1093/eurheartj/ehu002

43. Meral Kayikcioglu, Inan Soydan. Egg consumption and cardiovascular health. Arch Turk Soc Cardiol 2009;37(5):353-357

44. Robert A Koeth, Zeneng Wang, Bruce S Levison, Jennifer A Buffa, Elin Org, Brendan T Sheehy, Earl B Britt, Xiaoming Fu, Yuping Wu, Lin Li, Jonathan D Smith, Joseph A DiDonato, Jun Chen, Hongzhe Li, Gary D Wu, James D Lewis, Manya Warrier, J Mark Brown, Ronald M Krauss, W H Wilson Tang, Frederic D Bushman, Aldons J Lusis, Stanley L Hazen. Intestinal microbiota metabolism of L-carnitine, a nutrient in red meat, promotes atherosclerosis. Nat Med. 2013 May; 19 (5): 576-585. doi: 10.1038/nm.3145.

45. Zhu W, Gregory JC, Org E, Buffa JA, Gupta N, Wang Z, Li L, Fu X, Wu Y, Mehrabian M, Sartor RB, McIntyre TM, Silverstein RL, Tang WH, DiDonato JA, Brown JM, Lusis AJ, Hazen SL. Gut Microbial Metabolite TMAO Enhances Platelet Hyperreactivity and Thrombosis Risk. Cell. 2016 Mar 24;165(1):111-24. doi: 10.1016/j.cell.2016.02.011. Epub 2016 Mar 10.

46. Carol Johnston. Am J Lifestyle Med. Functional Foods as Modifiers of Cardiovascular Disease. 2009 Jul; 3(1 Suppl): 39S–43S. doi: 10.1177/1559827609332320.

47. Jane F Ferguson. Meat-Loving Microbes - Do steak-Eating Bacteria Promote Atherosclerosis? Cardiovascular Genetics. 2013:6:308-309. doi: 10.1161/CIRCGENETICS.113.000213.